Conjunctivitis (Pink Eye)

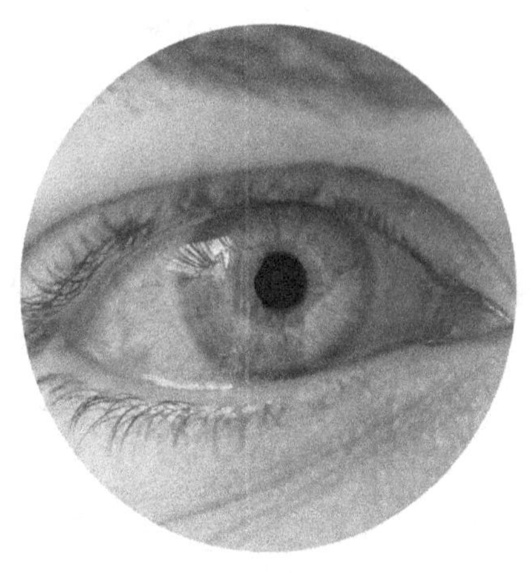

Dr. Sheila Harrison

Disclaimer

This content serves to provide general information about the disease and aims to empower you to seek prompt medical assistance if necessary to prevent complications. It's essential to stress that this information is not a substitute for consulting a qualified physician. The field of medical science is continually evolving, and due to the dynamic nature of medical knowledge, we recommend seeking expert advice if you encounter any inconsistencies or intend to take action based on the information in this content. Never disregard professional medical guidance or delay treatment based on something you've read online, including this material, or from any other online source. Always remember that the internet cannot cure you; rather, healing comes through the guidance of medical professionals and the providence of God.

Table of Content

Overview

A common infection of the eyes that results in inflammation of the tissues lining the eyelid (conjunctiva) is called pink eye. Allergens, irritants, germs, and viruses—including COVID-19, the coronavirus that causes the common cold—are the causes of it. Treatment options include eye drops, ointments, tablets, water flushes, and comfort care, depending on the reason.

Pink eye, also known as viral conjunctivitis, is a common, self-limiting illness that is usually brought on by an adenovirus. Herpes simplex virus (HSV), varicella-zoster virus (VZV), picornavirus (enterovirus 70, Coxsackie A24), poxvirus (molluscum contagiosum, vaccinia), and human immunodeficiency virus (HIV) are additional viruses that can cause conjunctival infection.

Being red in the eyes for 10 to 12 days after the commencement of viral conjunctivitis makes it extremely contagious. Patients should refrain from sharing towels, napkins, pillowcases, and other fomites, as well as from touching their eyes and shaking hands. Indirect eye contact with infected upper respiratory droplets, contaminated swimming pools, or inadvertent inoculation of viral particles from the patient's hands are the two ways that the virus might spread. Usually within two to four weeks, the infection clears up on its own.

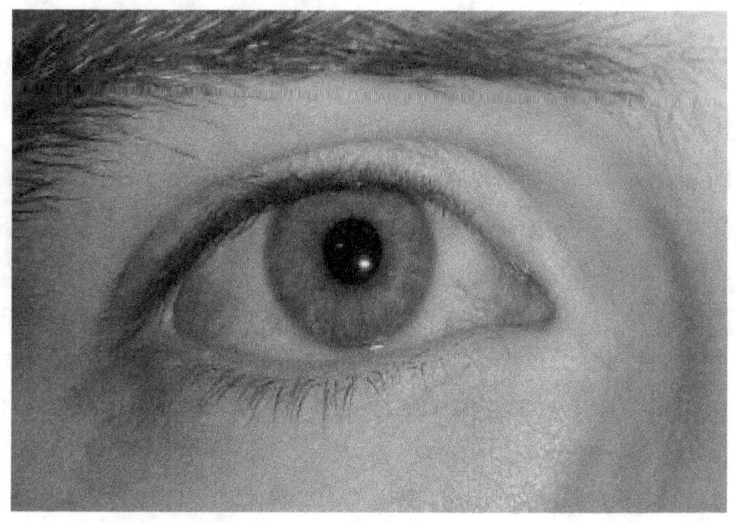

Section 1

Pink Eye (conjunctivitis)

A reddening or inflammation of the conjunctiva, the transparent tissue lining the outside and inner surfaces of your eyes, is known as pink eye. By keeping your eyeball and lid wet, this tissue assists. Viruses, germs, allergies, and other factors can all cause pink eye. Conjunctivitis is what is known medically as pink eye. One or both of your eyes may become pink.

How Pink Eye appears

The white portion of your eyes appears light pink to reddish, and your eyelids may be drooping or swollen. It is possible for you to notice crusting on your eyelids and lashes, or fluid (discharge) flowing from the infected eye.

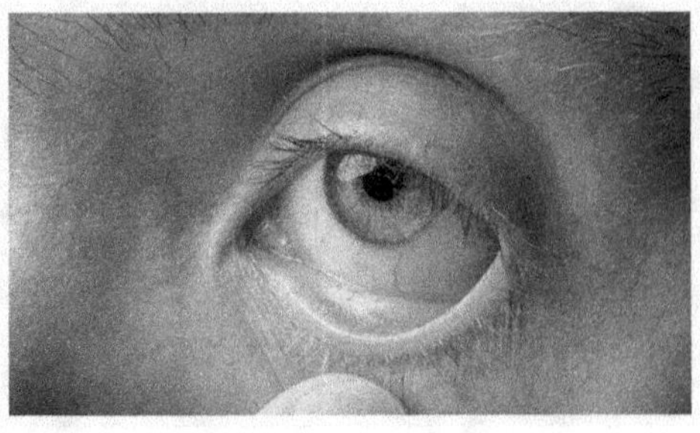

The distinction between pink eye and a stye

A stye and pink eye both have redness, sensitivity to light, and crusting around the eyelids as typical symptoms. However, there are differences between these two illnesses as well as different causes.

A stye is a painful, red bump that develops on your eyelid or inside it, usually on the edge of your lashes. An inflammation of the lining of your eyelid's inner surface and the outer layer of your eye is called pink eye. Your eyelid or the area around your eye does not get bumpy due to pink eye.

An infection in the oil glands on your eyelid is the source of styes. In addition to differentiating themselves from the causes of styes, viruses, germs, and allergies can also produce pink eye.

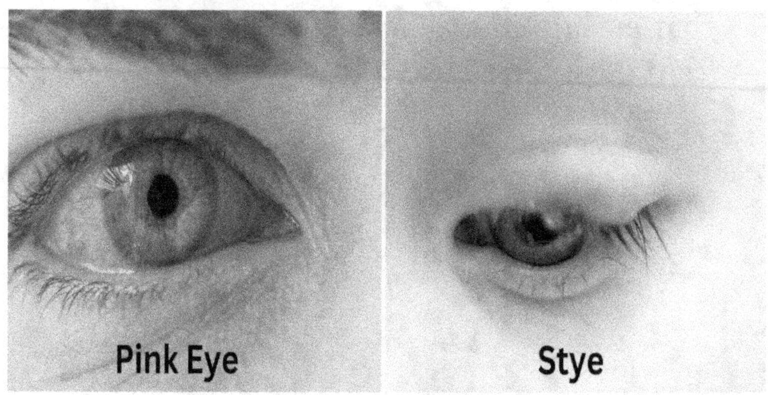

How common is pink eye?

One of the most prevalent illnesses of the eyes in both adults and children is pink eye. In the United States, there are over 6 million incidences of pink eye annually.

How to know if it's pink eye

Your healthcare professional is the only one who can provide a definitive diagnosis, however there are certain symptoms that are typical with pink eye that you should be aware of. If the white of your eyes is predominantly light pink to reddish, you most likely have pink eye.

- Is constantly tearing.
- Has a green, yellow or white discharge
- Itches.

Section 2
Symptoms and Causes

Symptoms of pink eye include:

- Redness in the white of your eye or inner eyelid.

- Increased tearing.

- Thick yellow discharge that crusts over your eyelashes, especially after sleep.

- Discharge: Green or white discharge from your eye.

- Gritty feeling in one or both eyes.

- Itchy eyes (especially in pink eyes caused by allergies).

- Burning eyes (especially in pink eyes caused by chemicals and irritants).

- Blurred vision.

- Increased sensitivity to light.

- Swollen eyelids.

Does pink eye spread easily?

Viral or bacterial pink eye is extremely contagious and spreads quickly from person to person. This is due to the fact that pink eye can spread before symptoms manifest. We all touch our eyes and faces far more often than we realize.

Allergy-induced pink eye is not communicable.

For what length of time is my pink eyes contagious?

If you have bacterial pink eye, you can spread the infection while you have the symptoms or for up to 48 hours after you begin antibiotic therapy.

For the duration of your symptoms, which are typically several days, if you develop pink eye from a virus, you are communicable. Pink eye might sometimes spread before any symptoms appear.

Section 3
Causes of Pink Eye

The pink or reddish hue of a pink eye is caused by inflammatory blood vessels that become more noticeable in the conjunctiva, the membrane that covers your eye. Inflammatory factors include:

- **Viruses:** The most frequent cause of pink eye is viruses. One type of virus that can cause pink eye is the coronavirus, which includes viruses like COVID-19 and the common cold.
- **Bacteria:** Staphylococcus aureus, Haemophilus influenzae, Streptococcus pneumonia, and Pseudomonas aeruginosa are common types of bacteria that cause bacterial conjunctivitis.
- **Allergens:** This includes allergens such as mold, pollen, or other things.
- **Irritating substances:** Shampoos, makeup, contact lenses, filth, smoking, and pool chlorine are examples of this.
- **Sexually transmitted infections (STIs):** STIs can be caused by bacteria (gonorrhea or chlamydia) or viruses (herpes simplex). Pink eyes can be brought on by STIs in both adults and infants.

- A foreign object in your eye.
- Blocked or incompletely opened tear ducts in babies.
- **Autoimmune conditions:** Pink eye is very rarely caused by diseases that make your own immune system overreact.

How Pink Eye is Spread

Pink eye spreads:

- when in close proximity to someone else—touching, shaking hands, etc. When you touch your eye, germs and viruses from someone else's hand go into yours.

- by coming into contact with surfaces that are infected with viruses or bacteria, then touching your eyes before cleaning your hands.

- By exchanging makeup that's tainted with viruses or bacteria, or by utilizing outdated eye makeup.

- Through having sex. When you contact infected semen or vaginal fluid and then touch your eyes without washing your hands beforehand, pink eye caused by STIs spreads.

Section 4
Diagnosis and Tests

Pink eye Diagnosis

Your child's or your own eyes will be examined by a pediatrician or ophthalmologist. Usually, your doctor can identify pink eye based on your medical history and symptoms. To examine your vision, you can perform an acuity test, often known as an eye chart test.

Speak with your doctor if you have:

- Had an infection, either bacterial or viral, recently.

- Allergies.

- Have you recently had anything irritating in your eye, such as chemicals or foreign objects?

- Received information about a sexually transmitted infection.

- Another reason to suspect you may have an autoimmune disease is a family history of the condition.

Clinical Exams to Diagnose Pink Eye

Testing may be recommended, even though it is uncommon, if your doctor believes that bacteria is the source of your pink eye or if the infection is severe. The area around your eye will be cleaned with a soft-tipped stick (swab), and the sample will be sent to a lab. Tests will be conducted in the lab to determine the cause of your pink eye.

How to distinguish between viral and bacterial pink eye

Your healthcare practitioner employs a few indicators to assist distinguish between bacterial and viral pink eye, even though the symptoms can be similar regardless of the cause:

- **Age:** Most adult occurrences of pink eye are caused by viruses. There are roughly equal numbers of pink eye infections in children caused by bacteria and viruses.

- **Ear infection:** It's typical for your child to have an ear infection at the same time they have bacterial conjunctivitis.

- **Amount of discharge:** An infection caused by bacteria is typically indicated by excessive discharge from the eye.

- **Color or tint of the whites of eye:** A salmon-colored (light pink) complexion could indicate a viral illness. A bacterial conjunctivitis is more likely to be reddish in color.

- **If it's in one or both eyes:** A virus is most likely the cause of your pink eyes if you have them in both of your eyes.

Section 5
Management and Treatment

Management

Adenoviral conjunctivitis is treated with supportive care. It is advisable to advise patients to apply cold compresses and lubricants, like cold artificial tears, for their comfort. For severe itching, topical vasoconstrictors and antihistamines may be used, although they are usually not recommended. Topical astringents or antibiotics can be used to avoid bacterial superinfection in susceptible patients. Clinical data supports the off-label prescription of topical ganciclovir for cases of epidemic keratoconjunctivitis (EKC), especially when corneal lesions are present. This is because topical ganciclovir is efficacious against at least Adenovirus serotype 8.

Virus-specific treatments

Topical antiviral medications, such as ganciclovir (Zirgan, Bausch & Lomb, Bridgewater, NJ), idoxuridine solution and ointment, vidarabine ointment, and trifluridine solution (Viroptic, Alcon, Fort Worth, TX), are typically used to treat patients with HSV-caused conjunctivitis.

To stop viral replication, high-dose oral acyclovir is part of the treatment for VZV eye illness.

Until the skin lesion is addressed, conjunctivitis linked to molluscum contagiosum will continue to worsen. Usually, the infection can be cured by removing the lesion's central core or by causing bleeding to occur inside the lesion.

Treatments

Treatment of pink eye depends on whether it's caused by bacteria, a virus, an allergen or something else.

Treatments for bacterial caused pink eye

In the event that bacteria are the source of your pink eye, your doctor will prescribe antibiotics (ointments, drops, or pills). Don't worry if applying ointment to your own or your child's eyes seems difficult. The ointment will probably melt into the eye if it goes near the lashes.

Treatment for virus-induced pink eye

Treatment is not necessary for viral pink eye unless it is brought on by the herpes simplex virus, varicella-zoster virus (shingles/chickenpox), or a sexually transmitted infection. Antiviral drugs are necessary for these infections since they are dangerous. They may leave your eye scarred or result in visual loss if left untreated.

A virus-induced pink eye cannot be treated with antibiotics.

Treatment for irritating substances-induced pink eye

Rinse your eyes for five minutes under a mild spray of warm water if something gets into them and irritates them. Steer clear of the irritating items going forward.

Four hours after you rinse your eyes, you should see an improvement. Contact your healthcare provider if they don't. Rinse your eyes with water and contact your healthcare practitioner right away if the material in your eyes is a strong acid or alkaline chemical (like drain cleaner).

Treatment for allergy-induced pink eye

Eye drops, either prescription or over-the-counter, are used to treat allergic conjunctivitis. These include anti-inflammatory medications like steroids or decongestants, or antihistamines to manage allergic reactions.

You might use a cold compress on your closed eyes to temporarily reduce your symptoms. By avoiding the allergens that trigger your symptoms or by using over-the-counter allergy medications, you can prevent this type of pink eye.

Treatment for sexually transmitted infections (STIs)-related pink eye

Though rare, STI-related pink eyes can be rather dangerous. Antibiotics are used to treat bacterial pink eye, just as they are for viral pink eye, and antiviral drugs are used to treat viral pink eye.

A dangerous kind of pink eye that can impair eyesight can strike newborns. Your unborn child may come into contact with the germs during delivery if you are carrying a STI. Every newborn's eyes are routinely treated with an antibiotic ointment in American hospitals to help prevent infection.

Treatment for autoimmune disease-related pink eye

Treating the underlying condition will also treat pink eye if it is caused by an autoimmune disease. To control your symptoms until your eye feels better, ask your healthcare practitioner.

Section 6

Medications for Pink Eye

Pharmacotherapy aims to avoid problems and lower morbidity.

1. Ocular Lubricants

These medications are used to treat symptoms.

Artificial tears (Altalube, GenTeal Tears, Bion Tears, Murine Tears, Nature's Tears) work to lengthen the time it takes for the tear film to break up and stabilize the precorneal tear film, which happens in dry eye conditions.

2. Antihistamines

These agents are used to treat severe itching.

- **Azelastine ophthalmic:** Azelastine competes with histamine for the H1 receptor and inhibits the release of histamine and other mediators involved in the allergic response.

- **Ketotifen, ophthalmic (Alaway, Zaditor, Zyrtec Itchy Eye Drops):** Ketotifen is a relatively selective H1 receptor antagonist and inhibitor of histamine release from mast cells. OTC.

- **Olopatadine ophthalmic (Pataday, Patanol, Pazeo):** Olopatadine is a relatively selective H1 receptor antagonist and inhibitor of histamine release from mast cells.

- **Corticosteroids:** Corticosteroids may be used for pseudomembranes and decreased vision and/or glare due to subepithelial infiltrates. They have anti-inflammatory properties and cause profound and varied metabolic effects. In addition, these agents modify the body's immune response to diverse stimuli. Extreme caution should be taken when using corticosteroids, as they may worsen an underlying HSV infection or induce dependency in the context of persistent EKC subepithelial infiltrates.

- **Prednisolone ophthalmic (AK-Pred, Pred Mild, Omnipred):** This agent decreases inflammation by suppressing migration of polymorphonuclear leukocytes and reversing increased capillary permeability. Less potent (eg, prednisolone 0.125%, fluorometholone 0.1%) are usually sufficient to treat subepithelial infiltrates. The steroid must be tapered very carefully, often over months. Topical cyclosporine A emulsion (Restasis, Allergan, Irvine CA) may provide a viable steroid-sparing alternative for selected patients.

- **Fluorometholone (Flarex, FML, FML Forte):** Fluorometholone inhibits edema, fibrin deposition, capillary dilation, phagocytic migration, capillary proliferation, collagen deposition, and scar formation. It decreases inflammation and corneal neovascularization, suppresses migration of PMNs, and reverses capillary permeability. It is believed to act by inducing phospholipase A2 inhibitory proteins.

- **Loteprednol ophthalmic (Alrex, Lotemax):** Loteprednol etabonate decreases inflammation by suppressing migration of polymorphonuclear leukocytes (PMNs) and reversing increased capillary permeability.

- **Immunosuppressant Agents:** Immunosuppressant agents are used as adjunctive or alternative treatment when steroid use is ineffective or requires minimization.

- **Cyclosporine ophthalmic (Restasis):** The exact mechanism of the immunosuppressive activity of cyclosporine is unknown, but preferential and reversible inhibition of T lymphocytes in the Go or G1 phase of the cell cycle has been suggested.

3. Antivirals

These agents are used for the treatment of HSV infection.

- **Trifluridine (Viroptic):** Trifluridine is a pyrimidine (thymidine) analogue drug of choice in the United States for topical antiviral therapy for HSV infection. It inhibits viral replication by incorporating viral deoxyribonucleic acid (DNA) in place of thymidine. It is prescribed initially 9 times per day until resolution of the epithelial keratitis, then QID for another week. If the patient has no response in 7-14 days, consider other treatments. Trifluridine requires refrigeration and contains the toxic preservative thimerosal.

- **Ganciclovir ophthalmic (Zirgan):** Ganciclovir is a selective antiviral activated only within infected cells by viral thymidine kinase. It is a viral DNA chain terminator and DNA polymerase inhibitor. It is available in gel formulation and is stable at room temperature. It is prescribed 5 times per day until resolution of the epithelial keratitis, then TID for an additional week.

- **Acyclovir (Zovirax):** This is a prodrug that inhibits viral replication; it is activated by phosphorylation by virus-specific thymidine kinase. The recommended dosage for acute epithelial keratitis or stromal keratitis ranges from 200 mg PO BID to 400 mg PO TID. Some clinicians recommend the highest anti-zoster strength of 800 mg owing to the variability among patients in gastric absorption and the resultant variability and unpredictability of measurable serum concentrations.

- **Valacyclovir (Valtrex):** Valacyclovir is a prodrug that is rapidly converted to the active drug acyclovir. It produces a greater serum concentration of acyclovir with smaller oral dosing. Valacyclovir is more expensive than acyclovir but can be as effective with a more convenient dosing regimen.

- **Famciclovir (Famvir):** This agent is a prodrug that, when biotransformed into its active metabolite, penciclovir, may inhibit viral DNA synthesis/replication. It has been used successfully in the suppression of genital herpes. Its efficacy in HSV keratitis currently is under study.

4. Antibiotics

Therapy must be comprehensive and should cover all likely pathogens in the context of the clinical setting. Antibiotics are used to prevent superinfections.

- **Ofloxacin ophthalmic (Ocuflox):** Ofloxacin is a pyridine carboxylic acid derivative with broad-spectrum bactericidal effect. It inhibits bacterial growth by inhibiting DNA gyrase. It is indicated for superficial ocular infections of conjunctiva or cornea due to susceptible microorganisms.

- **Trimethoprim/polymyxin B ophthalmic (Polytrim Ophthalmic Solution):** This combination is used for ocular infection of the cornea or conjunctiva caused by susceptible microorganisms.

- **Ciprofloxacin ophthalmic (Ciloxan):** Ciprofloxacin has activity against *Pseudomonas* and *Streptococcus* species, methicillin-resistant *Staphylococcus aureus* (MRSA), *Sepidermidis,* and most gram-negative organisms; it has no activity against anaerobes.

- **Sulfacetamide ophthalmic (Bleph 10):** This agent interferes with bacterial growth by inhibiting bacterial folic acid synthesis by competitively antagonizing para-aminobenzoic acid.

Section 7

Prevention of Pink Eye

Prevent the spread of a pink eye infection.

Due to its contagious nature, It's critical to stop viral conjunctivitis from spreading. Hands should not be placed in the infected or contralateral eye, and sharing of towels, linens, or cosmetics is discouraged. This goes for both the patient and the healthcare professional. It is best to urge infected patients to avoid going to work or school. It is advisable to advise contact lens wearers to stop using their lenses until all symptoms have subsided.

If you or your child has bacterial or viral pink eye, your healthcare provider may recommend staying home from work, school or daycare until you're no longer contagious. Check with your healthcare provider to find out how long that may be. You're usually less likely to spread the infection if you've been on antibiotics for 24 hours or no longer have symptoms.

Following good general hygiene and eye care practices can also help prevent the spread of pink eye.

- Don't touch or rub the infected eye(s).

- Wash your hands often with soap and water.

- Wash any discharge from your eyes twice a day using a fresh cotton ball. Throw away the cotton ball and wash your hands with soap and warm water afterward.

- Wash your hands after applying eye drops or ointment to your eye or someone else's eye.

- Don't share personal items such as makeup, contact lenses, towels or cups.

Section 8
Perspective / Prognosis

If I have pink eyes, what should I anticipate?

Pink eye is extremely contagious, yet it's usually not a serious condition. The majority of mild to severe episodes of pink eye resolve without medical intervention.

If the pink eye is severe, treatment is frequently required. It can spread the illness to others and reduce the duration of your symptoms.

Duration/Lifespan of pink eye

If you have conjunctivitis caused by bacteria, it should get better in a week. Even if your symptoms disappear, always take any medication as directed by your doctor.

Conjunctivitis caused by viruses often lasts four to seven days. The entire resolution process may take up to 14 days.

When to seek medical attention for pink eye

For pink eye, you don't always need to see a doctor. You can usually treat the symptoms at home until they go away on their own. However, you should never be afraid to contact your healthcare professional with any questions or concerns.

Certain symptoms may indicate a more serious issue, including an ulcer that could cause irreversible blindness. Make an immediate appointment with your physician or seek medical attention if you encounter:

- heightened light sensitivity, particularly in cases of extreme intensity.

- reduced vision or hazy vision.

- Eye pain.

- having the sensation of having something lodged in your eye.

- a lot of discharge coming from your eyes.

- Worsening symptoms.

Questions to ask your Doctor

- What's causing my pink eye?

- How can I relieve my symptoms at home?

- How do I use my prescription medication?

- How can I keep pink eyes from spreading?

- What new or worsening symptoms should I contact you about?

- Are there any requirements my child has to meet before returning to school/daycare?

Section 9
FAQs On Pink Eye

Does pink eye resolve itself?

In most situations, mild cases of pink eye resolve on their own in a matter of days to weeks. The majority of viral conjunctivitis causes are self-limiting. When treating bacterial conjunctivitis, antibiotics shorten the duration of your illness and your contagious period.

What quickly eliminates pink eyes?

The only way to eliminate pink eye more quickly is if germs are the cause. The duration of bacterial pink eye can be shortened with antibiotic eye drops. For other forms of pink eye, they are ineffective.

When can I go back to my regular life if I have pink eyes, such as going to school or working?

As soon as your symptoms disappear, you or your child can typically return to work, daycare, or school. This could occur two to seven days following a viral illness and up to 24 hours following antibiotic treatment for a bacterial infection.

Your eyes shouldn't have any:

- Yellowish discharge.
- Crusting on your eyelashes or in the corners of your eyes.
- Pink color.

When it's safe to return, make sure to consult your healthcare provider. You don't have to remain home if your pink eye was caused by an allergy or by something else that isn't communicable.

How can I lessen the discomfort caused by pink eye?

Since pink eye is often minor, you may typically manage its symptoms at home until they go away. Non-prescription "artificial tears" eye drops can help reduce burning and itching caused by irritants.

Note: Avoid using other types of eye drops as they could irritate your eyes. Do not use eye drops intended to relieve redness. If the second eye is not infected, do not use the same dropper bottle.

Additional actions you can do to alleviate pink eye symptoms include:

- Until your symptoms subside, cease wearing your contact lenses.

- Apply cool compresses to your eyes (or heated compresses if you prefer), and keep towels and washcloths separate from other people.

- To get rid of irritating materials, wash your face and eyelids with a light soap or baby shampoo and then rinse with water.

Will my pink eyes return?

Particularly if you have pink eyes from an allergy, pink eyes can recur. Your eyes may react each time you come into touch with an allergen—a material that causes allergies.

You may unintentionally re-infect yourself if you have bacterial or viral pink eye. In order to prevent contracting infectious pink eye again:

- Use hot water and detergent to wash your towels, washcloths, bed linens, and pillowcases. Replace them often.

- Till the illness clears up, avoid applying cosmetics on your eyes. Delete any makeup that was applied right before the infection began, as well as any outdated eye makeup.

- Put on glasses as opposed to contact lenses. Frequently clean your glasses.

- Disposable contact lenses should be discarded. Make sure all eyeglass cases and extended wear lenses are spotless. Only sterile contact solutions should be used. Hands-wash before putting in or taking out contact lenses.

- Don't use the same eye drops on a non-infected eye after using them on an infected one.

Conclusion

Typically, pink eyes are not significant. It is very curable and avoidable. Pink eye can go away on its own without treatment unless it is really severe. The best course of action is to take the required precautions to prevent contracting pink eye again or giving it to others. Always give your healthcare professional a call if you have any queries or concerns.